6 Minute Morning
Workout

6 Minute Morning
Workout

Faye Rowe & Sara Rose

Bath New York Singapore Hong Kong Cologne Delhi Melbourne

This edition published by Parragon in 2009

Parragon
Queen Street House
4 Queen Street
Bath BA1 1HE, UK

ISBN 978-1-4075-8131-6
Printed in Malaysia
Designed by Design Principals, Warminster

Photography: Ian Parsons
Models: Samantha Fuery, Jade, Louisa Jarvis
and Lucinda Jarvis

The publisher would like to thank the
following for permission to reproduce
copyright material: Ken Chernus/Taxi/Getty:
7; White Cross Productions/Photographer's
Choice/Getty: 12; iStockphoto: 17, 83 top

NOTE FOR THE READER
The views expressed in this book are those
of the author, but are general views and
intended as a guide only. Readers are
urged to consult a relevant and qualified
practitioner for specialized and tailored advice.
Appropriate independent advice should be
obtained from a medical practitioner before
carrying out any exercise, especially if you
haven't exercised before.

CONTENTS

INTRODUCTION

Keeping your body in tip-top condition doesn't have to mean spending hours in the gym. Just 6 minutes each morning, in the comfort of your own home, is all you need to keep yourself in shape.

Six minutes in the morning
It doesn't sound like a lot, but spending just 6 minutes each day working out is enough to turn you into a fitter, healthier person. If you want a toned body, flat stomach, well-shaped hips and thighs, and flexible limbs without spending hours in the gym, this is the book for you.

It's ideal for beginners, so the exercises won't come as a shock to the system.

No doubt you've picked up this book because you're finding it hard to make time for exercise. It's no surprise, considering the busy lifestyles most people lead these days, that your health gets shifted to the bottom of your "to do" list. The soaring cost of a gym membership, added to the fact that not many people have a gym on their doorstep (let alone one that doesn't cost the earth), means that the fitness-conscious among us are waking up to the idea of getting fit at home. The great thing about this book is that it covers such a wide range of exercises— and each section is easy to follow and fun to do.

As well as targeting your trouble zones, the stretching and toning sections offer an all-over makeover. So, even if your fitness goals change, this book will still be useful. An added advantage is that you don't need any bulky fitness equipment, so it won't take over the spare room and you won't have to break the household budget.

All the exercises in this book have been tried and tested by experts in the field and found to be very effective. They really do work, so let's get started!

The 6-minute concept

How easy would it be for you to devote 6 minutes in the morning to exercise? Even if you usually jump out of bed and dash straight off to work without time for breakfast, it's really not much of a sacrifice to make, especially when you consider the results you can achieve.

Six minutes is the average time it takes you to brush your teeth and have a wash, or to make a cup of coffee and eat a bowl of cereal. What we're trying to say is that, even if you're usually pushed for time in the morning, it won't be hard to negotiate a spare 6 minutes into your timetable. Even if you have to set your alarm clock a full 6 minutes earlier than usual, it's very unlikely to affect your quality of sleep or leave you tired during the day, so you won't feel hard done by. In fact, making time for exercise in the morning will give you a fantastic energy boost that should last all day. That's on top of a great new physique, which will really give you something to brag about.

Exercise is also known to boost levels of "happy hormones" (endorphins) in the brain, making you feel more cheerful and relaxed, with a higher sense of self-esteem.

Endorphins also beat stress, so you'll not only be a dream to work with, but you're also more likely to perform to your best abilities. And, when you're feeling optimistic, you're more likely to make healthy food choices, which will further help you to achieve your goals. Plus, since you'll get your workout done in the morning, it doesn't matter if you have to work late or fulfill social commitments in the evening—which you might be tempted to use as an excuse not to do your exercise routine.

An added bonus of exercising in the morning is that, since it's done on an empty stomach, you're more likely to burn fat reserves rather then simply work off food that's sitting in your stomach. It will also kickstart your metabolism, helping you burn more calories throughout the day—although that's not an excuse to eat an extra donut!

If you're naturally cynical, you might be wondering whether 6 minutes of exercise is enough to make a difference to your body. The good news is that it works. It's true that some fitness fanatics swear by hours of cardio for weight loss and fat burning, but studies have shown that spending a short time exercising at a high intensity (i.e. doing something that gets your heart rate pumping and makes you slightly out of breath) can be more effective than exercising at a moderate level for longer periods of time.

It's the good news we've all been waiting for and it's why we've created this handy book, so anyone with an interest in fitness can make a real difference to their body without it costing a fortune or having to spend hours working out in the gym. Now, all you have to decide is what you want to focus on each morning.

Four ways to fitness

This book is divided into four sections, each of which targets a common trouble zone or offers a total body workout. Each section is thoroughly explained later in the book, but if you don't yet know what you want to focus on, here is an insight into what each section can help you achieve.

Stretching

Targets: All the major muscles in the body—to make them longer, leaner and more toned.
What's involved: A series of challenging stretches that will leave your mind calm and your body more flexible.
Who it will suit: If you're stressed you'll benefit from this relaxing routine, but it's also great if you want to prevent your muscles from becoming bulky.

Body toning

Targets: Each of the major muscle groups in the body— it's an all-over workout.
What's involved: A wide variety of exercises that are fun to do, including squats, lunges, sidekicks, stepping, crunches, press-ups, and lifting dumbbells.

Who it will suit: People who want to see an all-over improvement in muscle tone and shape and who want to target the whole body instead of specific trouble zones.

Flat stomach

Targets: The four abdominal muscle groups that support your lower back, protect the internal organs, maintain your posture, and allow you to bend, twist, and sit up. They all look fabulous when trim and toned!

What's involved: Seated exercises such as knee lifts, and ones that you can do on the floor like pelvic tilts, plus a series of curls (mini sit-ups).

Who it will suit: Apple-shaped women (who tend to store fat around the middle) and new moms wanting to tone up saggy skin.

Hips and thighs

Targets: Like it says on the box, this section targets your hips, thighs and those stubborn pockets of fat around the tops of the legs that are so hard to shift.

What's involved: A series of squats, lunges, seated and standing exercises, plus a lot you can do lying on the floor.

Who it will suit: Anyone who struggles to shift fat from their lower half.

Warming up, cooling down

As with all forms of exercise, it's vitally important that you spend time warming up before you start and cooling down before you finish. Not only will it help prepare your muscles for exercise by making them more receptive, but it will also protect you from stiffness and injuries such as strains and cramp.

If you turn to pages 18–31, you'll find 14 easy exercises—nine warm-ups and five cool-downs—from which you can pick and choose in order to ease yourself in and out of the 6-minute plan. If you choose to do the hips and thighs, flat stomach or body toning plan, you should spend around 1 minute warming up and the same time cooling down. Make sure you carry out each warm-up exercise for no less than 20 seconds and each cool-down exercise for 10 seconds. Your body will thank you for it.

If you're doing the stretching plan, warming up and cooling down isn't necessary because the exercises in this section aren't strenuous enough to cause damage to the muscles. Instead, prior to the stretching plan, make sure you've had a brisk walk around your bedroom or a quick jog on the spot, because this will get the circulation going.

If you do feel any discomfort while carrying out any of the exercises, it's important that you stop what you're doing immediately and take a break. If you ever experience a nagging pain, or feel sick, dizzy or unusually out of breath at any time while doing the exercises, simply stop and book an appointment with your doctor to rule out any underlying health problems that might be causing the discomfort. It might put your workout plan on hold for a while, but it's best to be safe when it comes to your health.

If your muscles feel sore at any time (if you're not used to exercise, you're most likely to experience this during the first few days of doing the plan), then take some time out to rest until your muscles feel good enough to get going again. As long as you pick up from where you left off and finish the plan without any major disruptions, the effects will be the same.

If you're a complete beginner, you may want to ease yourself gently into the plan and do less repetition. That's fine if you do, just remember to be persistent and your efforts will pay off. Soon enough, you'll find that your body will be better able to cope with the routine and, when this happens, you'll know you've made amazing progress. Just stay positive, enthusiastic, and optimistic and you'll reap the rewards.

What to wear

Wearing the right kit can make a massive difference to your performance. What's vitally important is that you don't just roll out of bed and get

started while you're still in your pyjamas. Not only might this restrict your movement, but you could trip over baggy clothes, for example, and you won't be in the right frame of mind for exercise.

A breathable Lycra sports top or a fitted T-shirt coupled with stretchy leggings or shorts is the ideal combination. You can pick up some great gear in the sports shop but, if you're on a budget, an old pair of tracksuit bottoms and a fitted vest top should be just fine. The good news is that exercising at home means that you won't get spotted by friends or colleagues in less-than-flattering attire.

If you're exercising on carpet or in the garage, you can do so in trainers. Alternatively, if you're working out on a wooden floor or lino, make sure you stay barefoot to save you from slipping.

If you have long hair, tie back loose ends with a clip or headband to stop it hanging in front of your eyes—that way you'll be able to read this book and follow the plan without a problem.

What you'll need
Equipment: The great thing about this workout plan is that you don't need any expensive equipment. However, you could invest in a padded exercise mat to stop you from slipping, a stopwatch so you can accurately time the exercises, and some dumbbells that you feel comfortable

using (ask a shop assistant to help you choose a suitable starting weight). If you don't have the cash, a can of beans makes a good dumbbell because it's easy to hold.

Space: Make sure you clear a space that is big enough for you to move freely in—that means one where you can fully extend your arms and legs without hitting anything. This may involve a bit of furniture reshuffling, but clearing a space especially for exercise and using it every day means you're more likely to stick to the plan as you get used to the routine.

HOW TO USE THIS BOOK

If you're keen to make a start on getting a fabulous new body, it may be tempting to try to combine a few of the sections at once. However, we recommend that you stick to one section at a time and finish each two-week plan before moving on to another section.

This way, your attention will be focused on carrying out the exercises to the best of your ability, and you won't find yourself cutting corners or trying to achieve more than is necessary.

We recommend that, before you begin, you have a thorough read of the section you want to complete. This will help you familiarize yourself with the different exercises so you won't waste time wondering exactly how to do them when you start. Remember to spend time warming up, then move straight on to the 6-minute exercise plan and, once you've finished, on to the cool-down exercises.

The 7 day guide at the end of each section lists six exercises (with page references) that you should hold, or repeat (as directed), usually for 30 seconds. Once you've finished all six, simply repeat the routine to make it last for the full 6 minutes. It's as easy as that. These plans are a rough guide, so if you find any particular exercises tricky, feel free to replace them with something else. However, the closer you stick to the plan we've drawn up, the better you'll find the results will be.

We encourage you to stick to your chosen section (hips and thighs, flat stomach, body toning or stretching) for two weeks, because this is the perfect amount of time you will need in order to see results. If you make sure that you include occasional rest days, it's fine to run the plans one after another. The more you do, the better you'll look and feel.

Getting started

As with all exercise programs, it's important that you discuss this workout plan with your doctor before you start. This is important in order to rule out any health conditions that may prevent you from taking part. Hopefully, you'll be given the green light and a pat on the back, and then there'll be no stopping you!

Posture: Having good posture makes all the exercises easier to do and more effective, too. Good posture results from your spine maintaining its natural curve, without sagging. If your posture is incorrect, every movement you make will be inefficient, leading to weakness, aching joints and muscles, and an increased risk of injury.

Test your posture by standing on one leg—you should be able to balance without wobbling. Even if you do wobble, the good news is that certain exercises in this book, such as those in the body toning and hips and thighs sections, will naturally improve your posture because they strengthen the major muscles (the core muscles) that support your body.

The basic thing to remember is, if you're standing,

imagine your spine is extended beyond your head up toward the sky and that someone is pulling on the end to make you stand to attention, a bit like a puppet on a string. Make sure your shoulders are relaxed—an easy way to check is to roll them backward a few times. This will help you find their natural resting place.

Another point to watch out for is that your stomach muscles are "engaged" at all times, which basically means that they are pulled in, nice and tight. This will automatically prevent your back from curving, making the exercises more effective, and guarding you against injury. Make sure you bear all this in mind at all times when exercising.

Keeping elbows and knees soft: If an exercise requires you to extend your arms or legs, remember always to keep elbows and knees "soft" (slightly bent). It will prevent you getting injured.

Breathing: The correct way to breathe when exercising is to breathe in slowly through your nose (notice how your abdominal cavity rises as you

do so), and breathe out slowly through your mouth. Make sure you continue to breathe in and out regularly throughout. And don't hold your breath— this will cause your blood pressure to rise, which can be dangerous.

Lastly, keep a bottle of water close by—keeping hydrated means the muscles work better and you'll be less likely to get cramp. Now, you're set to go. Simply pick one of the four sections and begin!

Warm up/cool down

Warming up is essential before you begin any kind of strenuous physical exercise, to protect your muscles from strain. Likewise, cooling down helps the muscles relax and wind down after exercise.

WARM UP

Tempting though it is to save time by launching yourself
straight into an exercise routine, if you don't warm up
you are highly likely to injure yourself because cold
muscles and joints are less flexible and more prone to
strain. So the 6-minute routines do assume that you will
have done your warming up beforehand.

Hip circles

This exercise will mobilize your lower abdominal muscles.
Try to make sure that only your pelvis is rocking rather
than your torso.

1 Stand up straight with your knees
slightly bent, feet hip-width apart,
hands resting on your hips.

2 Tighten your abdominal muscles by
gently pulling your navel toward your
spine. This movement should feel light and
subtle—do not suck in your waist or hold
your breath.

3 Gently rotate your pelvis to the right
so that you are rotating in a full circle.

4 Repeat nine times to the right then
circle ten times to the left.

Waist twist

It's important not to move your hips and knees during this exercise, but do feel free to move your arms like a hula dancer if it helps you get into the right mood!

1 Stand up straight with your knees slightly bent (soft, rather than "locked"). Keep your feet hip-width apart and your hands resting on your hips.

2 Tighten your abdominal muscles by pulling your navel back toward your spine.

3 Keeping your hips and knees still, rotate your shoulders and head to the right, then return to the center.

4 Now twist to the left, rotating your head and shoulders and keeping your hips and knees still.

5 Repeat this exercise a further five times on each side.

1

Forward bend

With this exercise, bend only as far as is comfortable—you don't have to touch your toes. Remember, you'll be able to stretch farther as time goes by and you become more supple with exercise.

1 Stand up straight with your feet hip- width apart and your knees slightly bent rather than locked. Place your hands, palms downward, on the front of your thighs.

2 Tighten your abdominal muscles by gently pulling in your navel toward your backbone.

3 Slowly slide your hands down your legs toward your toes. Try not to overarch your back.

4 Position yourself so you feel a stretch in the hamstrings at the back of your legs but don't stretch so far that it hurts.

5 Hold for a count of three then return to the center (see step 1).

6 Repeat four more times. Keep your breathing steady throughout.

3

Side bends

Do not do this exercise quickly with your arms above your head as this will make it hard to control the movement.

1 Stand up straight with your feet hip-width apart, your knees slightly bent, and your arms by your sides.

2 Tighten your abdominal muscles by gently pulling your navel toward your spine.

3 Keeping your back straight and without leaning forward, slowly bend to one side from the waist so that your hand slides down the side of your leg. Straighten up again.

4 Repeat on the other side. Repeat four more times on each side.

3

FLATTER STOMACH IN A FLASH

A very simple way of making your stomach look flatter is simply to make sure your posture is correct. Good posture happens when your spine is in natural alignment rather than hunched or slouched. For an instant, more streamlined appearance, stand with your feet hip-width apart. Gently pull up through your legs, keeping your knees slightly bent. Lengthen your spine, pull in your stomach muscles, and stand tall. Keep your shoulders down and relaxed so that your neck is as long as possible. Before you know it—as if by magic, your stomach will look flatter!

Knee bends

This exercise loosens the hip flexor muscles and helps warm up all the leg muscles. Don't lock your knees as you do this, and bend only as far as is comfortable.

1 Stand with one hand resting on a support such as a high-backed chair or a table, your feet hip-width apart and slightly turned out. Tighten your abdominal muscles.

2 Slowly bend your knees and lower your hips, then straighten up again. Use your buttock and leg muscles to lower and straighten.

3 Repeat nine times.

Leg swings

This exercise warms up the hip joints. Don't swing your legs too high (about 45 degrees is high enough), and keep the movements controlled and flowing.

1 Stand with one hand resting on a support, such as a high-backed chair or a table, and balance on one leg with the knee slightly bent. Tighten your abdominal muscles to protect your back.

2 Gently swing your other leg forward and backward. Keep your hips still as your leg moves from back to front. Swing up to 20 times on one leg then swap sides and swing on the other leg.

WATCH POINT

Never point your toes inward while exercising—this can damage your knees.

2

Standing quad stretch

1 Stand up straight with your feet
hip-width apart and your knees soft
(slightly bent). Tighten your stomach
muscles to protect your back.

2 Bend one leg up behind you and hold
your foot or ankle with your hand.

3 Hold for 5–10 seconds then release
and repeat on the other side.

4 Repeat twice more on each leg.

Marching

This warming-up exercise will help
to raise your body temperature and
increase blood flow to the muscles.
March on the spot for at least a minute,
swinging your arms and gradually
raising your knees higher as you go
(but not so that you're goose-stepping).
Make sure your breathing is deep and
regular as you march. Once you feel
warm, take the time to perform a few
stretching exercises.

Standing hamstring stretch

1 Stand up straight with your knees hip-width apart and your knees soft (slightly bent).

2 Extend one foot forward so that it is pointing in front of you with the weight resting on its heel. Tighten your abdominal muscles to protect your back.

3 Rest your hands on the thigh of the bent leg to support your body weight.

4 Bend forward from the hip and feel the stretch in the back of the thigh of the straight leg.

5 Hold for 5–10 seconds then release and repeat on the other side.

6 Repeat twice more on each leg.

4

COOL DOWN

As well as helping to prevent dizziness and a sudden drop in body temperature (which can make you feel unwell), cooling down realigns working muscles to their normal position to avoid post-exercise tightness and stiffness. It also helps you to relax and gives you a few quiet moments to yourself before carrying on with the rest of your day. Cooling-down stretches can be held for longer than 10 seconds because the muscles are warm.

Lying full body stretch

1 Lie flat on your back and relax. Breathe in and extend your arms outward and backward so that they meet behind your head. Try to keep your arms on the floor throughout the movement but if this isn't possible just keep them as low as you can.

2 Gently stretch out your body from your fingertips to your toes. Your lower back may lift from the floor a little.

3 Hold for a count of 20 then slowly release, bring your arms back down to your sides, and relax.

WATCH POINT

If you have any back problems, keep your knees bent slightly throughout. Also be aware that, if you are unused to stretching, you may feel tightness in your shoulders or cramp in your feet—in which case, relax. You will be able to hold this stretch for longer with practice.

2

Leg lift and cross

1 Lie on your back with your legs out straight and your arms stretched out to the sides.

2 Breathe in to prepare, and tighten your abdominal muscles. Lift your right leg up to the ceiling as you breathe out, and flex your foot.

WATCH POINT

If you can't take your foot all the way to the floor, bend your arm up to meet your foot, and rest the foot on your hand.

2

3 Using your abdominal muscles to control the movement, lower your leg across your body over to the left side until the foot touches the floor.

3

4 Hold for a count of 20 then slowly return to the starting position. Repeat on the other side.

Knee hug

2

1 Lie on your back with your legs straight. Tighten your abdominal muscles and pull both legs up to your chest.

2 Take hold of your knees and hug your knees tighter to your chest. Hold for a count of ten.

3 Release the pull then repeat as many times as you wish.

Hip and thigh stretch

1 Kneel with one knee above the ankle and foot flat on the floor, and stretch your other leg behind you so that the knee touches the floor.

2 Place your hands on your front knee to balance yourself. Hold this position for a count of ten then repeat on the other leg.

WATCH POINT

Be sure to pull in your abdominal muscles during the whole of the hip and thigh stretch in order to protect your back.

2

Standing full body stretch

1 Stand tall with your arms by your sides and your feet hip-width apart.

2 Raise your arms above your head and clasp your hands together.

3 Stretch your arms up as high as possible and feel the stretch in your arms, chest, stomach, hips, and thighs. Hold for a count of ten, then release.

3

2 Stretching

Stretching is an excellent way to keep your body in shape. Not only is it soothing, it will help your muscles to stay flexible and protect them from injury. It will also help you look longer and leaner.

INTRODUCTION

Stretching every day not only counters the muscle-shortening effects of exercise, it can work wonders for your mind, too. Many fitness trainers recommend their clients take up stretching once they've hit a plateau with exercise because it develops the muscles in a different way to cardio or other weight-based exercise.

The best thing about stretching is that it'll make you look longer and leaner. Plus, this section will prove that you don't have to jump up and down in order to streamline your silhouette.

This section is perfect if you have an existing medical condition such as asthma, and you are unable to do more strenuous forms of exercise. However, some of the stretches will make you slightly out of breath, so concentrate on keeping your breathing steady.

The benefits
Soothing music is ideal to accompany stretching exercises, and this routine will help calm your mind for the day to follow —it's almost like meditating. Physically, stretching will help tone and lengthen your muscles and it will also make you more flexible. Doing it regularly will help reduce the risk of injury to the joints, muscles and tendons while exercising, and it's a great way of relieving any soreness or tension you feel after a gruelling workout.

Stretching is also a great way to stimulate the lymphatic system, which in turn helps to cleanse the body of toxins and boost circulation. So, it's a great way to kickstart a detox and help keep cellulite at bay.

WATCH POINT

It can be tempting to "bounce" while in a stretch—for example, if you're trying to push yourself while reaching for the floor. However, this can strain the muscles so avoid it at all costs.

Effective stretching

The 18 stretches in this section aim to stretch out each of the major muscle groups—the thighs, bottom, calves, ankles, stomach, waist, arms, shoulders, chest, back, and neck. Each stretch lasts for around 30 seconds and you should aim to hold each stretch for three sets of 10 seconds, with a brief pause in between. In order to make the routine effective, it's important that you don't stop for more than a minute between exercises. Like all exercise, stretching has cumulative effects, so keep going!

What you'll need

For this routine you'll need a non-slip mat and a chair, and for some exercises you'll need to be near a wall for support. You don't need to spend one minute warming up or cooling down to do this workout, but take a brisk walk around your room or jump up and down on the spot for a few seconds to make sure you're warm.

Once you've got used to the routine, if you feel you can increase certain stretches, do so slowly and gently by moving further into position. Just remember to take your time and not to push yourself. You'll be amazed at how far you can go when you put the practice in and you'll be lithe and limber in no time at all.

NOTE

If you ever develop a persistent pain by doing any of the stretches in this routine, see your doctor for advice.

THIGHS AND LEGS

Seated hamstring stretch

The hamstrings are the muscles running up the backs of the thighs to your bottom. It's common for people to suffer with tight hamstrings, especially if they do a lot of sport, which is why it's great to stretch them out. If you don't stretch, tight hamstrings can cause the hips and pelvis to rotate backward, resulting in bad posture.

1 Sit down on the floor with your legs straight out in front of you, keeping your feet flexed. Sit up straight so your back isn't hunched and place your hands on your hips.

2 Lean forward from the hips, letting your upper body drop down toward your feet. You can extend your arms and try to touch your toes, although if you do this, make sure that you don't curve your back.

3 Hold for 10 seconds but don't bounce. Return to the starting position and repeat twice more.

2

Inner thigh stretch

This stretch targets the muscles in the inner thighs, which are called the adductors. It's an easy way to stretch both the legs at once and is great if you combine it with a short meditation.

1 Sit on the floor with knees bent and soles of your feet pressed together so you're in a "frog" position. Hold the soles of your feet together with both hands.

2 Sit up, so your back is straight, and pull your stomach muscles in toward your spine.

3 Using the muscles in your inner thighs, push your knees down

toward the floor. Make sure you don't bounce your knees.

4 When you've got your knees as far as you can go, hold the stretch for 10 seconds. Slowly release, then hold for two more sets of 10 seconds.

WATCH POINT

Make sure you don't curl your back. It makes it easier to reach the floor, but you'll be making the stretch less effective.

Hip flexor stretch

This stretch targets the hip flexors (the iliopsoas muscles) as well as the muscles at the front of the thighs. It may feel like a small movement but it works really well at easing away the tension in the muscles that may have built up if you've been sitting down for most of the day.

1 Stand with feet hip-width apart and hands resting on your waist.

2 Extend your right leg directly out behind you by about a foot (30cm). Keep both feet flat on the floor.

3 Bend both knees so your whole body drops down toward the floor by a few inches (5cm).

4 Letting your heel naturally lift off the floor, tilt your pelvis forward, bringing your bottom forward, and your hips up. You should immediately feel the stretch in the hip and the front of the thigh of the extended leg.

5 Hold the stretch for around 7 seconds, gently release then hold for another 7 seconds. Repeat with the left leg.

4

Quadriceps stretch

The quadriceps muscles are found at the front of your thighs and are often referred to as the "quads." Depending on how flexible you are, this stretch may feel quite hard to do at first but it quickly becomes easier. If, on the other hand, you need to feel a bigger stretch, simply thrust slightly forward the hip of the leg you are stretching.

1 Stand at a right angle to the back of a chair and hold the back with your right hand for support.

2 Keeping your knees together, bend your left leg backward, grab your left foot or ankle with your left hand, and bring your heel toward your bottom. Make sure you keep your right leg straight, with the knee soft (not locked) and your right foot flat on the floor.

3 Hold the stretch for around 7 seconds, slowly release, then hold for another 7 seconds. Repeat with the right leg.

WATCH POINT

Don't allow your knees to drift apart while you're holding the stretch, or you won't be targeting the quads effectively.

3

BOTTOM

Bend and stretch

This stretch targets all the muscles at the back of the thighs and in the bottom. Look toward the toes of your extended leg while you are doing the stretch, because it will inspire you to go as far as you can.

1 Stand a large step away from the front of a chair, with feet hip-width apart.

2 Lift your right leg and rest your right foot firmly on the seat of the chair. Your hands should be on your hips.

3 Bend over from the waist, and reach out to touch the toes of your right foot with both hands. You should feel the stretch in your right buttock and thigh.

4 Hold for two sets of 7 seconds on your right leg, without bouncing, and then repeat with the left leg.

3

WATCH POINT

Make sure that the chair is in the right position— you don't want the foot of your extended leg to be dangling off the edge.

Seated gluteal stretch

This is a great way to stretch out the muscles in your bottom, while sitting on it! It's quite a hard move to perfect, but the deep, intense stretch will give great results.

1 Sit on the floor with your back straight to create a good posture.

2 Extend your right leg straight out in front of you, keeping your foot flexed.

3 Bend the knee of your left leg and bring it toward you so your left foot is flat on the floor.

4 Cross your left foot over your right leg, so your left foot is level with your right knee.

5 Take your right arm and hug your left knee. Pull it toward your right shoulder until you feel the stretch. Your body should be twisted from the waist. Look to the left.

6 Hold for two sets of 7 seconds, and then repeat with the other leg.

WATCH POINT

To get the best stretch you can, don't lean back. Keep your back straight and the stretch will be more effective.

5

Cross and dip

This stretch targets the same muscles as the Seated gluteal stretch, but it will also develop your balance. The stretch will get easier as your calves become more flexible, because you'll be able to lower yourself down further without letting your foot rise up off the floor.

1 Stand behind a chair at a right-angle to it with feet hip-width apart and knees soft. Hold on to the back of the chair with your left hand for support.

2 Bend your right leg and bring your right foot across to meet your left leg, so it's resting above your left knee.

3 Slowly bend the knee of your left leg and lower yourself down toward the floor. Your left foot should remain flat on the floor at all times.

4 As you go down, your left knee should push your right foot higher into the air, which is when you should start to feel the stretch in your right hip, buttock, and top of thigh.

5 Once you've gone down as far as you can, hold the stretch for two sets of 7 seconds. Repeat with the other leg.

WATCH POINT
Keep your back straight at all times; it will stop you from getting a bad back.

3

CALVES & ANKLES

Runner's calf stretch

If you do a lot of running or walking you may find that your calves feel tight and inflexible. This stretch will help them feel loose and tension-free.

1 Get down on the floor on your hands and knees, with your knees resting directly below your hips and your hands below your shoulders. Curl your toes under so they are resting on the floor.

2 Push up off the floor with both hands and straighten your legs, pushing your bottom into the air. Your elbows and knees should be soft.

3 Try to lower your heels gently to the floor. Hold for three sets of 10 seconds, returning to the start position in-between.

WATCH POINT

This is quite a difficult stretch and you may not be able to hold it for the full 10 seconds at first. Just try your best and don't give up.

2

Push-off calf stretch

You usually see joggers doing this stretch before a big run—that's because it's a really good way of performing a controlled calf stretch that targets the gastrocnemius muscle (the big muscle at the back of the calf). To get the best stretch possible, make sure your full weight is shifted toward the wall.

1 Stand at arm's length from the wall, with your feet shoulder-width apart.

2 Extend your right leg out in front of you and bend your right knee.

3 Place the palms of your hands, at shoulder height, flat against the wall.

4 Take one step back with your left leg and, keeping it straight, press your heel firmly into the floor. You should feel the stretch in the calf of your left leg. Keep your hips facing the wall and your rear leg and spine in a straight line.

5 Hold the stretch for two sets of 7 seconds, then repeat with the other leg.

4

WATCH POINT

If you want to feel a greater stretch, simply move your extended leg a little bit further away from the wall.

Point and flex stretch

This is a really easy stretch to do and it may remind you of having dance classes as a child. It's best to keep doing the movement explained below rather than holding the stretch for a set period of time. Make sure you put the effort into really pointing and flexing the feet—the further you go, the better the stretch.

1 Sit on the floor with both legs stretched out in front of you. Sit upright with your back straight and your hands resting on the floor by your bottom for support.

2 Start by flexing your feet toward you as far as you can get them. Then, point them away from you down to the floor as far as you can.

3 Keep repeating the movement slowly until the 30 seconds are up.

WATCH POINT

Try not to rush the movement. Your priority is to feel the stretch rather than do as many repetitions as you can in the time allowed.

2

STOMACH & WAIST

Push down

The Push down is a great warm-up for the stomach and waist. It's a really gentle movement that helps to get you warm, while stretching out your major muscles.

1 Stand with feet hip-width apart and your hands resting by your sides. Make sure your legs are straight with knees soft.

2 Lean to the right, sliding your right arm down your right thigh toward your knee as you go. Keep your back straight and your head and neck in line with your spine at all times. You should feel the stretch in your left side.

3 Hold for two sets of 7 seconds, returning to the starting position in-between, then repeat on your left side.

2

WATCH POINT
You don't need to tilt over very far, just aim to touch the side of your knee with your hand.

Up and over

This exercise is an old-style way of targeting the muscles at the side of your waist, which are called the obliques. It's a great way of stretching out your love handles and it also helps you to feel really refreshed in the morning.

1 Stand with feet hip-width apart and your hands resting by your sides. Make sure your legs are slightly bent with knees soft. Keep your back straight and your head and neck in line with your spine.

2 Raise your left arm over your head and lean over from the waist to the right, so that your right hand travels down the side of your right leg. Your left arm should be reaching up and over your head. You should feel the stretch in the left side of your waist.

3 Hold for two sets of 7 seconds then slowly return to the starting position and repeat on the other side.

1

2

WATCH POINT

Don't try to stretch down too far—just do enough to feel it working.

ARMS, SHOULDERS & CHEST

Shoulder stretch

This is an easy stretch to do, and will really get your shoulders loosened up. It's great to do if you've been particularly stressed-out recently, because it will help to get rid of any built-up tension.

1 You can do this stretch from either a standing or a seated position. Extend your right arm directly out in front of you so it's parallel with the floor.

2 Using your left hand, grip the back of your right arm between your elbow and your shoulder and use it to bring your right arm gently across the front of your chest. You should feel the stretch down the inner side of your right arm and across your right shoulder blade.

3 Hold the position for two sets of 7 seconds and then repeat with the other arm.

WATCH POINT

Stop yourself from rotating by making your hips face forward at all times.

Pec stretch

Your pectoral muscles (pecs) are the big muscles that sit under your bust. Stretching them out will help get rid of any knots or tension that may have built up from carrying heavy bags. Plus, this stretch will help encourage deep breathing, which will enable you to feel a whole lot perkier and more refreshed in the morning.

1 Stand with feet hip-width apart. Place your palms on your lower back then gently pull your shoulders back together and stick your chest out until you feel the stretch. Keep your elbows soft.

2 Hold the stretch for three sets of 10 seconds.

WATCH POINT

When you bring your shoulders back, be careful not to arch your back. All the movement should come from the shoulders.

1

Inner arm stretch

This targets all the muscles in your upper arms—you'll be surprised at how easy it is to feel the stretch.

1 Stand in an open door frame, with your abs tight and body straight.

2 Hold on to the door frame with your left hand just below shoulder level, or as high as is comfortable. Take a big step forward so your left arm is extended out behind you. Keeping your hips facing forward and your head and neck in line with your spine, rotate your upper body to the right until you feel the stretch in your left arm. Lean forward to feel a greater stretch.

3 Hold for two sets of 7 seconds then turn around, step forward and repeat the stretch with your right arm.

WATCH POINT

Don't worry if you find it difficult to get your arm up to shoulder height because you can still achieve a good stretch by having it slightly lower.

Tricep stretch

Your tricep muscles are found at the back of the top of your arms. Giving them a good stretch will boost circulation and help to get rid of any blotchy, pimply skin that may reside there.

1 Stand with feet hip-width apart. Lift your right arm above your head and bend your elbow so your hand drops down behind your neck.

2 Grip your right elbow with your left hand and pull it gently to the left—this will automatically force your right hand to dip down between your shoulder blades. You should feel the tricep muscle stretch in your right arm. Keep your chin lifted, so you don't put a strain on your neck.

3 Hold the stretch for two sets of 7 seconds then repeat the stretch, working your left arm instead.

2

WATCH POINT

This movement makes it really easy to let your head fall forward so your chin is resting on your chest, but don't let this happen because it will put a strain on your neck. Keep your chin lifted and eyes forward throughout the stretch.

BACK & NECK

Upper back stretch

Stretching out the muscles in the back will have a therapeutic effect on both your body and your state of mind. The back is one of the first areas to retain tension and stress, so stretching out the muscles will help to put you at ease and set you up for the day ahead.

1 Stand with feet hip-width apart. Interlink your fingers and push your hands out in front of you as far as possible. Your palms should be facing away from you.

2 Allow your upper back to relax by lowering your shoulders to their natural resting position.

3 Hold for 10 seconds. You should feel the stretch between your shoulder blades. Pause for a brief moment, then repeat the stretch twice more.

WATCH POINT
If you find it hard to get your back to relax, just take a deep breath and lower your shoulders. This will have an instant relaxing effect.

2

Lower back stretch

This stretch is ideal for targeting the muscles across your lower back, which have a tendency to ache, especially if you've had a bad night's sleep. Stretching them in the morning will help to reduce your risk of injury during the day.

1 Stand with feet hip-width apart and knees slightly bent.

2 Place your hands on your inner thighs with your palms facing outward.

3 Engage your abdominals and slowly arch your spine until you feel a stretch across your lower back.

4 Hold for around 8 seconds then slowly stretch up through the spine until you are back in a normal standing position. Keep your back straight, with your chin up and looking forward.

5 Repeat the stretch three times.

WATCH POINT

If you're not feeling the stretch, simply move your palms further down your thighs—this should help to increase it.

3

7 DAY PLAN

This 7 day plan is an example of the way you can structure your stretching regime, which should be repeated for a further week, making a two-week schedule. We've chosen a mixture of different stretches to target each of the major muscle groups in the body to give you a great all-over program.

You'll do two sets of six stretches each morning to last for 6 minutes. If you want to draw up your own plan you can. However, we recommend you start with our plan and monitor your results—how flexible you become and how relaxed you feel—then you can adapt it if you need to. Now, let's get started…

Day 1

Seated hamstring stretch p36
Seated gluteal stretch p41
Runner's calf stretch p43
Push down p46
Pec stretch p49
Upper back stretch p52

Day 2

Inner thigh stretch p37
Seated gluteal stretch p41
Push off calf stretch p44
Up and over p47
Inner arm stretch p50
Tricep stretch p51

Day 3

Hip flexor stretch p38
Cross and dip p42
Push off calf stretch p44
Up and over p47
Shoulder stretch p48
Lower back stretch p53

Day 4

Quadriceps stretch p39
Bend and stretch p40
Point and flex stretch p45
Pec stretch p49
Upper back stretch p52
Lower back stretch p53

Day 6

Quadriceps stretch p39
Hip flexor stretch p38
Cross and dip p42
Push off calf stretch p44
Inner arm stretch p50
Lower back stretch p53

Day 7

Seated hamstring stretch p36
Bend and stretch p40
Push off calf stretch p44
Push down p46
Tricep stretch p51
Upper back stretch p52

Day 5

Seated hamstring stretch p36
Seated gluteal stretch p41
Runner's calf stretch p43
Up and over p47
Inner arm stretch p50
Lower back stretch p53

3 Body toning

Toning your body will increase your muscular strength and improve your overall physical fitness. Having a trim, toned physique also makes you look good and can do wonders for your self-confidence.

INTRODUCTION

Having a trim, toned physique makes you strong and healthy looking. Plus, building a bit of muscle will boost your metabolic rate, so you'll burn more calories during the day and reduce the amount of fat that your body stores. A good body-toning regime is an excellent, low-impact way to exercise, and can be a great stress reliever, too.

The exercises in this section focus on the legs, buttocks, stomach, arms, chest and back, so each day you'll have a thorough workout. Some parts of the body, such as the buttocks and thighs, are harder to tone, which is why you'll find more exercises devoted to these areas in the plan.

If you find any of the exercises difficult to do, you can replace them with something else and adapt the program. Similarly, if you feel your arms are toning up much faster than your legs, make a few substitutions and get back to it.

BOOST YOUR BODY TONING

Making small changes to your lifestyle and the way you eat can help boost the effects of the plan and maximize your results. Try the following tips for healthy eating and living, but remember to speak to a doctor or nutritionist before making changes to your diet.

- Cut down on saturated fat and refined sugar, found in convenience foods like cakes, cookies, sweets and fast food.
- Stick to pure, fresh foods such as vegetables, fruit and wholegrains.
- Combine lean protein with vegetables or salad at mealtimes.
- Drink up to eight glasses of water a day to help flush toxins from your system.
- Be more active—take the stairs instead of the lift and try to walk everywhere you can.

The benefits

When the two weeks are up, you may find that your clothes feel looser and that your muscles look more defined. How well you respond depends much on your body composition—if you naturally have more muscle mass, then you're likely to respond quicker. If you want to look more toned in time for a special occasion, follow the "boost your body toning" tips (above) alongside the exercise program, because they will help you to achieve your goals.

Effective toning

Some exercises in this section require you to repeat the movement until the full 30 seconds are up. We've given the suggested number of repetitions you should try, but just do as many as you can comfortably achieve in that time. To make it effective, it's important that you don't stop for more than a minute between exercises. Shorter recovery periods result in better muscles all round and improved muscle endurance. So keep going!

What you'll need

For this routine you'll need a non-slip mat, a set of dumbbells (or cans from the cupboard), a chair, a sturdy step (like the bottom of a staircase). You'll also need to use a wall for some exercises. Don't forget to warm up and cool down!

LEGS

Standing calf raises

The calf muscles are hard to target, although studies have shown that walking in high heels can help to tone them up! To get really sexy, shapely calves, we recommend you try this exercise instead.

1 Stand with both feet near the edge of a raised object such as a stair or a big chunky book. Place the ball of your right foot on the edge of the raised object, letting your heel extend off the edge.

2 Hold on to a wall or a chair for support and, lifting your left leg into the air slightly by bending at the knee, gently let your right heel drop down until you feel the stretch in your calf. Keep your back straight, your head up, and your right leg straight.

3 Rise up on to your right toe as high as you can and hold for a second while flexing the calf muscle.

4 Carefully return to the starting position, then repeat with the left leg.

5 Aim to do around ten repetitions on each foot.

2

WATCH POINT

Ensure that you don't slip off the raised object by carefully controlling the move.

Squat

The Squat is one of the most effective exercises for toning the muscles in the legs and buttocks, including the hamstrings (at the back of the legs). Plus, it's a great way to build strength in the lower body. It's an easy exercise to get right and you can really feel it working.

1 Stand with feet hip-width apart. You can either place your hands on your hips or hold on to the back of a chair for support if needed.

2 Look straight ahead and count to three while you bend your knees and push your bottom out behind you, until you feel the muscles working in the backs of your thighs and buttocks. The deeper you can squat, the better it is for working those muscles, but make sure you keep your feet flat on the floor at all times. Keep your back straight and make sure your spine is in line with your head and neck.

3 Return to the starting position, counting to three as you go, and get ready to do it all over again!

4 Aim to do around ten repetitions.

2

WATCH POINT

Make sure your feet remain flat on the floor. Don't let them rise up when you bend your knees.

Step-back lunge

This exercise will help to tone the quadriceps (known as the quad muscles) at the front of your thighs to give you a healthy and athletic look.

1 Stand with feet hip-width apart and rest your hands on your hips.

2 Keep your right foot firmly on the floor and lunge backward with your left leg, bending your knee until it rests around 6 inches (15cm) above the floor. You should be balancing on the ball of your left foot, and will be able to feel the muscles working in the front of the left thigh.

3 Return to the starting position, then repeat with the other leg.

4 Aim to do around three on each leg, or more if you feel comfortable.

2

WATCH POINT

Check behind you to make sure you have enough room to step back into the lunge. If you want to make the exercise more demanding, you can hold dumbbells as you do it.

Side kick

The Side kick is an energetic exercise that will get your heart rate pumping and really burn some calories. It's great for toning the hamstrings and quads and it will give your waist a workout too.

1 Stand with feet hip-width apart. Bring your hands up to your chest and form loose fists, while keeping your elbows bent and by your sides to help you balance.

2 Raise your right leg off the floor and kick it out to the side in a swift, controlled move. Be careful not to flick your leg, as you could jar your knee or hip.

3 Bring your leg back to the starting position and repeat the movement for 30 seconds.

4 Repeat the movement with your left leg.

5 Aim to do around ten on each leg.

WATCH POINT

Be careful that you don't use too much force to shoot your leg out to the side or you may end up straining a muscle or jarring your knee.

2

BUTTOCKS

Lunge

Lunging is great for strengthening and toning the muscles and is a firm favourite among personal fitness trainers.

1 Stand with feet hip-width apart. Rest your hands on your hips or by your sides.

2 Step forward with your right leg, bending your knee so your thigh is almost at a right-angle to the floor. Your right foot should be flat on the floor. Your left leg should be slightly bent at the knee and the ball of your left foot should be resting on the floor behind you, with your heel slightly in the air.

3 Hold for a second, then push off the floor with your right foot and return to the starting position.

4 Repeat the movement with alternate legs until the 30 seconds are up.

5 Aim to do around ten lunges (five on each side) in the allotted time.

2

WATCH POINT

Don't rush the lunge or go down too far or you'll end up banging your knee on the floor. Always make sure you go at your own pace.

Crane stand

This exercise is like the Superman, but standing up. It's great for working your buttocks, hamstrings and lower back but it does take a lot of skill and balance to achieve, so do it slowly for best results.

1 Stand on your left leg and take a few seconds to find your balance.

2 Extend your left arm out in front of you and your right leg out behind you. Try to keep your right leg as straight as possible without locking the knee.

4 Gently straighten up from the waist so you're back in the starting position. Repeat with the opposite arm and leg.

5 Aim to do around four, or more if you feel comfortable.

3 Reach out as far as possible and tilt your body over from the waist so your left arm drops down to the floor.

WATCH POINT

This exercise is suitable for everyone. Just concentrate and take it slowly to make sure you keep your balance.

Side-step squat

This exercise is an 80s aerobics classic, which is so effective that it's still used today in most good fitness routines. Squatting to the side targets all the muscles along the inner thigh and bottom to help sculpt a beautiful-looking rear view.

1 Stand feet hip-width apart, with your feet slightly turned out and flat on the floor. Rest your hands on your hips or by your sides.

2 Step your right leg out to the side and bend your right knee, so you lower yourself by several inches a (few centimeters) toward the floor. Let your full body weight fall onto your right leg. Keep both feet firmly on the floor at all times.

3 Push off from the floor with your right foot and return to the starting position.

4 Repeat the movement with your left leg and keep repeating the exercise on alternate legs until the 30 seconds are up.

5 Aim to do around ten on each leg.

2

WATCH POINT

Doing the full warm-up routine at the start of this book will help you avoid pulling the muscles in your groin as you do this exercise.

Stepping

This is a great exercise if you like "feeling the burn," Stepping up on to a stair forces the glutes (the muscles in the buttocks) to squeeze and contract, so will help create a pert bottom.

1 Stand at the bottom of the stairs or in front of a big chunky book. Rest your hands on your hips or let them rest by your side.

2 Step up on to the step with your left leg and let your right leg follow.

3 Step down off the step with your left leg and let the right leg follow.

4 Repeat, starting with the right leg.

5 You should be able to manage around 15 or more during the 30 seconds.

2

WATCH POINT

Do this barefoot or wear a good pair of sports trainers rather than slippery socks for this exercise so that you don't slip off the step. Plus, don't rush the move.

STOMACH

Plank

This doesn't sound or look too taxing but, if you do it right, you'll find that it's one of the most intense exercises in the book, and very effective at toning the abdominal muscles.

1 Lie on the floor on your front, resting your forehead on the backs of your hands.

2 Keeping your elbows bent, slide your hands across the floor, rotating from the shoulders, until you find your perfect "press-up" position either side of your chest.

3 Curl your toes underneath you and push up off the floor with your hands. Keep your elbows soft to stop them locking, and keep your neck and head relaxed and in line with your spine.

WATCH POINT

This exercise can be difficult to do so don't over-strain yourself—you may be able to hold the position for only five seconds at first. Just persevere!

4 Hold the pose for 10 seconds, then gently lower yourself back down to the floor again. Remember to breathe during the exercise.

5 Start by doing three sets of 10 seconds. Try to increase the time that you hold the Plank to the full 30 seconds by the end of two weeks.

3

Reverse curl

This is great for targeting the stomach muscles. You should feel it really working all across your stomach—the harder you concentrate, the more effective it will be.

1 Lie on the floor, making sure that the small of your back is pressed against the floor and not arching upward. An easy way to do this is to engage your abdominal muscles so you feel them contract.

2 Bring your knees toward your chest and cross your feet at the ankles. Rest your hands by your sides on the floor for support.

3 In one carefully controlled move, use your stomach muscles to lift your bottom and lower back off the floor. Aim to straighten your feet and knees and push them up toward the ceiling. You don't have to move far, just enough to feel your muscles working.

4 Count to two on the way up and two on the way down.

5 When you've done 30 seconds' worth of repetitions, place your feet back on the floor. Return to your starting position.

6 Aim to do around seven during the 30 seconds.

WATCH POINT

Make sure you're lying on soft carpet or a padded exercise mat to reduce the risk of bruising your spine.

3

Waist twist

Make sure you have a lot of space around you so that when you swing your arms you don't hit anything. This is a fun exercise to do and it really gets to work on the obliques (the muscles at the side of your waist), to help define a curvy silhouette.

1 Stand with feet hip-width apart, hands by sides, and knees slightly bent.

2 Extend your arms out in front of you and form loose fists with both hands.

3 Swing your arms from side to side, making sure your feet stay firmly on the floor, and your hips face forward. Start off slowly and then build up speed, making sure you keep control of the movement and your hips stay facing the front.

4 When the 30 seconds are up, drop your arms back down by your sides and return to the starting position.

5 Do as many as you can in the 30 seconds.

3

WATCH POINT

Don't get carried away while swinging your arms as you may end up pulling a muscle. If you have to go slowly to control the movement, so be it.

Crunches

This is an intense workout for your stomach muscles and a great way of getting a washboard-flat tum.

1 Lie on the floor, knees bent and feet (apart) flat on the floor in line with your hips. Make sure your lower back is pressed into the floor. Put your hands behind your head to support your neck.

2 Engage your stomach muscles, by pulling your abdominals toward your spine, and lift your upper body off the floor as far as you can without arching your lower back. You may find that you can't get up very high, but it's the effort of moving that counts, so make sure that you're pushing yourself as hard as you comfortably can. With practice, you may be able to sit up completely.

3 When you can't go any further, pause for 1 second. Then gently lower yourself back down into the starting position and repeat.

4 Do as many sets of five as possible, with a brief rest between. By the end of two weeks you should aim to do the Crunches continuously for 30 seconds.

WATCH POINT

Don't use your neck to pull yourself up or you'll feel the strain the next day. Supporting your neck with your hands will prevent this, but don't use your hands to lift your head off the floor—let your stomach muscles do all the work.

3

ARMS

Press-ups

This is a good all-round exercise for toning the major muscles in the arms. It's really good for developing upper-body strength and balancing out a pear-shaped figure.

1 Lie face-down on the floor, with your forehead resting on the backs of your hands. Slide your hands around to rest at shoulder level, to find your ideal "press-up" position either side of your chest.

2 Use your arms to lift your upper body off the floor and bring your knees in toward your chest a little so they're resting on the floor, taking most of your body weight. Cross your feet at the ankles and raise them off the floor slightly. This should automatically cause your body weight to shift back on to your arms.

WATCH POINT

Engaging your tummy muscles will help keep your back straight and reduce any risk of injury.

3 Bend your elbows and gently lower your upper body back down to the floor, keeping your head and shoulders level and in line with your spine at all times. Then push off the floor with your hands, raising your upper body into the air. Aim to get your arms straight, while keeping your elbows soft. Repeat this movement.

4 Aim for two sets of ten during the 30 seconds.

3

Bicep curl

The biceps are the muscles at the front of the upper arms. They are relatively easy to tone, so practising this exercise will help give you shapely arms that you'll want to show off.

1 Stand up tall with feet hip-width apart and knees soft.

2 Extend your arms out in front of you with palms facing upward, holding a can of soup or a dumbbell in each hand.

3 Bend your elbows and bring both your hands in toward your shoulders so that your arms form right-angles.

4 Reverse the movement so that your elbows are fully extended in front of you again. Keep your elbows soft at all times.

5 Repeat the movement until the 30 seconds are up.

6 Aim to do as many as you can during the time period without rushing.

3

Bench dip

As well as working your triceps, this will help improve your core stability and tone up your tummy. It's especially great for the arms because you're using your body weight to strengthen and tone.

1 Sit on the edge of a chair with your hands resting either side of your bottom, gripping the edge of the seat.

2 Walk your feet away from the chair as far as you can so your bottom comes off the edge of the chair.

3 Letting your arms take your body weight, bend your elbows and, with knees bent, slowly lower your body toward the floor—make sure you don't end up sitting on the floor; hovering just above the floor is the ideal position. Make sure your weight is evenly distributed so you don't topple the chair.

4 Straighten your arms, so you bring your lower body back up. Repeat Steps 3 and 4.

5 Aim to do around six.

WATCH POINT

Keep your forearms vertical at all times—it will help to reduce the amount of strain on your shoulders.

Circles in the air

This exercise is great for general toning of the arms and shoulders. Using weights will also help to develop strength in the arms and have a pumping effect on the muscles, so you'll look great in short-sleeved tops.

1 Stand with feet hip-width apart, knees slightly bent and arms resting by your sides.

2 With a dumbbell in each hand, cross your arms in front of each other level with your hips, then circle them up toward the ceiling so they cross over in the air above your head. Then bring them back round to the starting position.

3 Pause for a second then repeat the movement in the opposite direction.

4 Aim to do around 15 in the 30 seconds.

3

WATCH POINT

Keep your arms fully extended as you circle them so you are working as many muscles as possible, but remember to keep your elbows soft.

CHEST

Wall push-up

This is like a standing press-up and is great for toning the muscles in the chest, especially the pectoral muscles, which can be found underneath your bust.

1 Stand around two feet away from the wall with feet hip-width apart and legs straight. Make sure your knees are soft.

2 Lean forward and place your palms flat against the wall.

3 Bend your arms at the elbows and bring your chest toward the wall.

4 Squeeze the muscles in your chest and push off from the wall so you are standing back in the start position.

5 Aim for around 15 during the 30 seconds.

WATCH POINT

Make sure you really put some effort into pushing off from the wall—that way it will work your arms as well as your chest. If you master the move, it will help you to achieve a perky bust!

Prayer

This is excellent for toning the pectoral muscles. Like the Wall push-up exercise, toning these muscles will help to give you a more youthful-looking bust.

1 Either while standing or sitting, press the palms of your hands together at shoulder height while extending your elbows out to the sides.

2 Hold the pose for as long as you can—ideally around 10 seconds, pressing your palms together with as much force as you feel comfortable with. Take one second to rest and then repeat the pose for 30 seconds.

3 Aim to hold the pose for 10 seconds and then take 1 second to rest and start again. By the end of two weeks you should aim to hold the pose for the full 30 seconds.

WATCH POINT

Many people will find their joints crack when doing this exercise, so start by pressing the palms lightly together and gradually start to build up the pressure. Doing the exercise this way will help prevent you from getting cramp.

1

7 DAY PLAN

This plan is an example of the way you can structure your exercise regime, which you can repeat for a further week, making a full 14 day fitness program. We've chosen exercises to target each of the major muscle groups in the body to give you a great all-over workout.

Each morning you will start with a brief warm-up. We've picked six different exercises each day to create a 3-minute routine, which should be carried out twice to make the workout last a total of 6 minutes.

You can easily draw up your own plan if you want to. Make sure you include a good mix of exercises but, if you want to aim for weight loss as well as toning, remember that the standing exercises will burn a lot more calories than the others. Plus, any exercise that targets the legs is going to create a big calorie expenditure. Only you can know your body's major trouble zones, so can include extra exercises to target those particular areas.

We recommend you start with our plan and monitor your results. Now, let's get started.

Day 1

Squat p61
Side kick p63
Crane stand p65
Reverse curl p69
Press-ups p72
Bench dip p74

Day 2

Standing calf raises p60
Lunge p64
Stepping p67
Plank p68
Bicep curl p73
Prayer p77

Day 3

Step-back lunge p62
Crane stand p65
Waist twist p70
Crunches p71
Bench dip p74
Wall push-up p76

Day 4

Lunge p64
Stepping p67
Waist twist p70
Bench dip p74
Circles in the air p75
Prayer p77

Day 5

Standing calf raises p60
Side-step squat p66
Crunches p71
Press-ups p72
Bicep curl p73
Wall push-up p76

Day 6

Step-back lunge p62
Side kick p63
Stepping p67
Plank p68
Circles in the air p75
Prayer p77

Day 7

Squat p61
Standing calf raises p60
Side-step squat p66
Reverse curl p69
Press-ups p72
Bicep curl p73

4 Flat stomach

Toning up your stomach muscles improves your posture and helps protect your back from injury. A flat stomach is also flattering and will enhance your figure, whatever you choose to wear.

INTRODUCTION

Most of us would love to have a flatter stomach but just can't face the thought of hours of strenuous sit-ups. But the key to a flatter stomach is to exercise little and often. Doing the quick, easy routines in this section will give you a flatter stomach in two weeks.

The benefits
Apart from the obvious benefit of improving your appearance, firming and toning up your stomach muscles will improve your posture and balance, and increase your flexibility. Building muscle tone doesn't happen overnight, but the beauty of this short routine is that you won't become bored or burned out. Keep it up and you'll have a tighter tum in two weeks.

Effective exercising
Some exercises in this section require you to repeat the movement until the

full 30 seconds are up. Just do as many reps as you can comfortably achieve in that time. To make it effective, it's important that you don't stop for more than a minute between exercises. Shorter recovery periods result in better muscles all round and improved muscle endurance. So keep going!

What you'll need
For this section you'll need a chair, a non-slip mat, a cushion, and a pillow or towel to support your head and neck.

Don't forget to warm up and cool down!

EATING FOR A FLAT STOMACH

Adopting a few healthy eating tips can help beat bloating and boost the effects of exercise. Don't ever skimp on liquids if you think it could ward off bloating because drinking lots of water actually promotes a flat stomach by flushing toxins from your system and curbing your appetite. If your body feels starved of water then it will hold on to what there is, which can lead to water retention and the appearance of bloating.

Drink at least eight glasses a day, but don't drink a lot before exercise because it will put pressure on your bladder. You'll know you're well hydrated by checking the color of your urine—the paler it is, the better.

Stomach muscles explained

It helps to have a basic idea of which muscles you need to work on to make your stomach appear flatter.

There are four abdominal muscle groups, which form a natural corset around the middle. They support your lower back, protect internal

organs, and enable you to bend, twist and sit up. The deepest of the abdominal muscles is the transversus abdominis, which wraps horizontally around your waist and keeps your lower back stable. The rectus abdominis runs from the pubic bone to the bottom of the ribcage. This muscle enables your trunk to bend and is important for maintaining your posture.

The external and internal obliques run up the sides of your body and enable you to bend to the side and twist your spine. The exercises in this section will work to strengthen all these muscles for a firmer, flatter, fabulously toned stomach.

SEATED EXERCISES

These easy exercises are great for a quick tummy-toning session and for postural realignment. You'll need a straight-backed, sturdy chair—not one on castors.

Seated stomach workout

This tones and flattens your deep stomach muscle (transversus abdominis) and the one that runs down the front of your stomach (the rectus abdominis).

1 Sit forward on a chair. Keep your feet flat on the floor, hip-width apart, with your knees over your ankles and your palms on your thighs.

2 Sit up straight. Tighten the abdominal muscles by gently pulling your navel in toward your spine. Hold for 10 seconds, then relax.

3 Rest for a count of three before doing any repetitions.

4 Aim to do around two to four.

WATCH POINT

Remember to breathe regularly as you do this exercise—don't hold your breath because it will make your blood pressure rise, which can be dangerous when exercising.

Seated knee lift

This seated exercise will work your rectus abdominis—the muscle that runs down the front of your stomach. Make sure your movements are controlled and flowing.

1 Sit on the edge of a chair with your knees bent and pressed together and your feet flat on the floor. Hold on to the sides of the chair, then tighten your stomach muscles.

2 Lean back slightly and lift your feet a few inches off the ground, keeping your knees bent and together.

3 Slowly pull your knees in toward your chest and curl your upper body forward. Then lower your feet to the floor. Rest for a count of three before you do any repetitions.

4 Aim to do around six.

3

WATCH POINT

Don't lean too far forward or you'll fall off the chair!

CONTROLLING YOUR MOVEMENTS

Make sure that all exercises are performed slowly, carefully, and with your full attention. You really do need to concentrate on what you're doing and think about how your body is responding to any exercise. If an action hurts or you do it quickly, then you're not doing it properly. Movements should flow in a gentle, controlled manner. This enables your muscles to stretch naturally.

PRONE EXERCISES

Exercising in this position means you are working against gravity, making your muscles work even harder. Remember to keep your elbows soft, not locked.

Belly tightener

This shortens the abdominal muscles, which is good for posture and creates the appearance of a flatter stomach.

1 Kneel down on all fours with your hands shoulder-width apart, your elbows slightly bent and your knees under your hips. Keep your head in line with the rest of your body and look down at the floor, making sure that your chin isn't tucked into your chest.

2 Relax your abdominal muscles then slowly draw in your navel toward your spine.

3 Hold the muscles in for a count of ten then slowly relax. Breathe slowly and steadily throughout this exercise.

4 You should aim to do around two to four.

WATCH POINT

Pull up the abdomen by using your deep abdominal muscles, not by arching your spine.

Easy plank (tension hold)

Holding your body in a three-quarters plank shape strengthens the deep transverse muscles that cross the stomach area. Keeping your knees on the floor makes this exercise much easier than the traditional plank, which you can progress to when you feel ready.

1 Adopt a traditional press-up position but keep your knees on the floor and your feet in the air. Your fingers should point forward, your elbows stay straight but not locked, your head should be in line with your body and your feet together. Keep your shoulder blades drawn into your back and make sure you don't dip in the middle or raise your bottom in the air.

2 Hold this position for a count of ten, breathing regularly throughout.

WATCH POINT

Avoid this exercise if you have shoulder problems. If you feel any strain in your back muscles, move your knees further apart.

3 Aim to do around two.

1

PELVIC TILTS

These exercises tighten the abdominal muscles without putting any strain on your back. They're a simple way to tone and strengthen your abdominal area.

Simple pelvic tilt

This easy exercise is particularly good if you're trying to shape up post-pregnancy.

1 Lie on your back with your knees bent and feet flat on the floor, hip-width apart, and your spine in neutral (see below). Rest your arms by your sides, with your palms facing the floor, and tighten your abdominal muscles.

2 Press your lower back down into the floor and gently tilt your pelvis so that the pubic bone rises, then tilt it back down.

3 Repeat several times, using a slow, steady rhythm.

4 You should aim to do around eight to twelve.

KEEPING YOUR SPINE IN NEUTRAL

This is the correct position for your spine during exercise. Lie down on your back, flat on the floor with your knees slightly bent and feet hip-width apart. Place your thumbs on your bottom ribs and your little fingers on the top of the hip bones. Draw these two points together by gently pulling your navel toward the floor to tighten your abdominal muscles. Keep your back in contact with the floor and do not arch your spine.

Lower abdominal raise

This is a harder exercise that will really work your deep abdominal muscles. If it seems easy then you're not doing it properly!

1 Lie on your back with your knees bent, feet flat on the floor and hip-width apart. Make sure your spine is in neutral. Keep your arms by your sides with the palms facing upwards.

2 Lift your legs into the air at an angle of 90 degrees to your body.

3 Tighten your abdominal muscles and slowly lower one foot to the floor then bring it back up again. Then repeat this exercise using the other leg.

4 You should aim to do around six to eight.

3

2

BASIC CURLS

These exercises will tone the rectus abdominis muscle, which runs down the front of your stomach. As you lift your head and shoulders, this muscle contracts at both ends. Avoid these exercises if you have neck problems.

Abdominal curl

Say farewell to sloppy sit-ups—a few properly executed curl-ups will work wonders in helping you achieve a flatter stomach.

1 Lie on your back with a firm, flat pillow or a small towel underneath your head. Keep your feet hip-width apart, parallel and firmly on the floor, and your knees bent. Rest your hands on your thighs.

2 Set your spine to the neutral position and tighten your abdominal muscles.

3 Flex your spine to lift your head and shoulders gently about 30 degrees off the floor. Your hands will slide up toward your knees as you curl. Keep your lower back in contact with the floor at all times. Slowly curl back down in a continuous movement.

4 You should aim to do around six.

2

Moving curl

This exercise gives your rectus abdominis an intensive workout by repeating the hardest part of the abdominal curl.

1 Lie on your back with your feet flat on the floor, knees bent and your arms by your sides (palms facing downwards). Keep your spine in neutral.

2 Tighten your abdominal muscles. Start curling up by lifting your head and shoulder blades off the floor while reaching forward with your arms.

3 Curl up about 30 degrees. Then extend your arms and lift and lower yourself just a few inches up and down from this position.

4 Repeat several times, then lower.

TOP TIPS FOR GREAT CURLS

- Always keep your knees slightly bent (flexed).
- Breathe out as you curl up and breathe in on the return.
- Never hold your breath when exercising—blood pressure will rise and this can be dangerous.
- Perform all exercises in a slow, controlled manner.
- Don't put your hands behind your neck because you are likely to tug on the neck vertebrae.

5 You should aim to do around two to four.

3

OBLIQUE CURLS

Twisting curls work your rectus abdominis muscles and the obliques, the muscles that give definition to the waist. These exercises will tighten your stomach muscles and trim your waist.

Basic oblique curl

1 Lie on your back with your knees bent, feet flat on the floor and hip-width apart. Put your hands by your temples at the sides of your head.

2 Lift your left leg and rest the ankle of that leg across your right thigh—this will turn your supported left leg out slightly. Keep your spine in neutral and tighten your abdominal muscles.

3 Curl up, rotating your trunk to the left and breathing out as you do so. Your right elbow should be moving toward your left knee. Keep your left side in contact with the floor to help support your back.

4 Curl back down again, breathing in as you do so, then repeat this exercise to the other side using the other leg.

5 You should aim to do around six to eight.

REVERSE CURLS

Reverse curls give a good workout to the transversus abdominis, the deepest abdominal muscle that wraps around your waist, and the rectus abdominis, the stomach muscle that's responsible for the six-pack look.

Reverse curl

Remember not to arch your back as you do this exercise.

1 Lie on your back with your spine in neutral, your arms by your sides, palms facing downward. Tuck your knees in toward your stomach and cross your ankles.

2 Tighten your abdominal muscles by gently pulling your navel in toward your spine.

3 Roll your knees toward your chest and then lower them down again.

4 You should aim to do around six to eight.

1

3

WATCH POINT

Remember to breathe regularly throughout.

ADVANCED CURLS

These exercises are not for absolute beginners. You should tone your abdominal muscles with a few weeks' worth of routines before you attempt these exercises.

Double-leg push-out

This exercise works the transverse (deep) abdominal muscles as you extend your legs.

1 Sit on the floor with your knees bent and your feet parallel, toes just touching the floor but your heels lifted off it.

3 Extend both legs in front of you but do not straighten your legs completely. Bring them back to the starting position.

2 Lean back slightly and support yourself by placing your hands behind you, palms downward. Tighten your abdominal muscles.

4 You should aim to do around ten.

Pillow roll

This exercise tones and strengthens your obliques and is a safe way to mobilize your spine. Your shoulders and arms should stay on the floor but you may find to begin with that the opposite arm and shoulder come up slightly.

1 Lie on your back on the floor with your arms out to the sides at shoulder height, palms flat on the floor. Keep your knees bent. Your feet should be touching and off the floor but to make this exercise easier you can keep your feet on the floor if necessary.

2 Put a cushion or pillow between your knees—this will make you keep your knees together, which is important for this exercise.

3 Tighten your abdominal muscles and remember to breathe normally—do not hold your breath.

4 Slowly bend your legs toward the floor on your right side, rolling your head to the left. Feel each part of your body peel up as you move—your buttocks, then hips, then waist and ribs. Keep going until your right knee and foot are touching the floor with your left leg lying on top.

2

5 Move your knees and head back to the central position.

6 Repeat this exercise on the other side with your legs toward the left side and your head to the right.

7 Aim to do six on each side.

Leg lift

This exercise helps to develop the deep (transverse) abdominal muscles as well as working your hamstrings (the muscles at the back of your thighs).

1 Lie on your back with your arms by your sides, palms facing downward. Keep your knees bent and feet hip-width apart, flat on the floor. Tighten your abdominal muscles.

2 Raise your left leg to the ceiling, keeping your knee slightly bent, then lower it. Then raise your right leg and lower it in the same way.

3 Aim to do around ten for each leg.

SETTING THE PACE

The aim of a toning program is to make your muscles work harder, either by increasing the time you exercise or by increasing the intensity of your workout. Your muscles will start to become tired during the last repetitions and you may feel a burning sensation in the area you're working but this is normal and will pass as soon as you rest. Muscle soreness and stiffness is highly likely in the beginning, particularly if you're new to exercise, but if you can hardly move then you've overdone it. Rest up for a day or so and start again at a reduced intensity.

2

Leg stretch

This exercise tests your balance as well as working your stomach muscles.

1 Lie on your back on the floor with your feet hip-width apart and your knees bent. Breathe in to prepare.

2 As you breathe out, tighten your abdominal muscles and pull one knee at a time up to your chest.

3 Breathe in and grasp your left knee with both hands.

4 Breathe out and slowly straighten your right leg up to the ceiling, keeping your back and your shoulders on the floor at all times.

5 Breathe in and bend the right leg back into your chest. Repeat the exercise with the other leg.

6 You should aim to do around ten for each leg.

WATCH POINT

If you feel your back arching, raise your extended leg higher to flatten it out.

STRETCHES

Your exercise routine concentrates on working your abdominal muscles hard to shorten them but it's important to remember that these muscles also need to be stretched in order to keep your body supple and injury-free.

Cobra stretch

This modified yoga position is excellent for stretching your stomach muscles.

1 Lie on your front on the floor and put your hands underneath your shoulders.

2 Breathe in to prepare, then gently push your arms up until they are straight but your elbows are not locked. This will lift your head and chest upward and you will feel a stretch in your abdominal muscles. Your hips should stay in contact with the floor throughout.

3 Hold for a count of ten then lower yourself back to the ground.

WATCH POINT

Stretch only as far as is comfortable or you may strain your back muscles.

Sitting body twister

1 Sit on the floor with your legs straight out in front of you. Bend your left leg and cross it over your right knee.

WATCH POINT

Stretch only as far as is comfortable.

2 Gently rotate your trunk and head toward your right as far as is comfortable, keeping your buttocks on the floor throughout.

3 Hold for a count of ten then release and return to the starting position. Repeat on the other side.

Side stretch

1 Kneel on your left knee and straighten your right leg out to the side.

2 Put your left hand on the floor and bring your right arm over your head until you feel a stretch in your side.

3 Hold for a count of ten then return to the starting position. Repeat on the other side of the body.

TOP TIPS FOR SUPER STRETCHING

- Only stretch warm muscles.
- Slowly ease the muscle into position.
- Do not bounce into position.
- Never overstretch—mild discomfort is acceptable but if it hurts, you should stop.
- Don't hold your breath—breathing freely will enable blood to flow to the muscles.

2

Standing waist stretch

1 Stand with your legs fairly wide apart, knees soft. Turn your right foot outward and bend the knee of the right leg so that you can lunge to that side. Keep your left leg straight with the foot flat on the floor and pointing forward. Rest your right palm on your right thigh to support your body weight.

2 Lift your left arm above your head and lean toward your right side. Hold for a count of ten. Repeat on the other side.

WATCH POINT

Don't lean too far over — you should feel a stretch in your obliques but it shouldn't hurt.

7 DAY PLAN

Here's a simple plan for you to follow, which should be repeated for a further week, making a full 14 day fitness program. Although these exercises are grouped into 6-minute sessions, if you're new to exercise please don't feel you have to start off doing the whole routine—you can build up the amount of time you spend and the types of exercises you do. You can also make up your own routines.

Do what feels right for you

The exercise program outlined on these pages suggests that you do one 6-minute routine every day. However, if you do not usually exercise regularly it is a good idea to start off by doing the routines every other day to give your body time to recover. Similarly, if you experience stiffness or pain the day after exercising, it is important to take a break that day. Each routine should take 6 minutes to do, but this may vary depending on the amount of reps you do. The exercises in this book will tone your stomach muscles quickly, but be aware that they are not for fitness or weight loss.

Day 1

Belly tightener p86
Simple pelvic tilt p88
Abdominal curl p90
Pillow roll p95
Cobra stretch p98
Standing waist stretch p101

Day 2

Seated stomach workout p84
Seated knee lift p85
Easy plank p87
Lower abdominal raise p89
Cobra stretch p98
Side stretch p100

Day 3

Simple pelvic tilt p88
Basic oblique curl p92
Reverse curl p93
Leg lift p96
Sitting body twister p99
Side stretch p100

Day 4

Abdominal curl p90
Double-leg push-out p94
Pillow roll p95
Leg stretch p97
Standing waist stretch p101

Day 5

Seated stomach workout p84
Moving curl p91
Double-leg push-out p94
Leg lift p96
Cobra stretch p98
Standing waist stretch p101

Day 6

Belly tightener p86
Lower abdominal raise p89
Reverse curl p93
Pillow roll p95
Sitting body twister p99

Day 7

Easy plank p87
Simple pelvic tilt p88
Moving curl p91
Basic oblique curl p92
Leg stretch p97
Cobra stretch p98

Hips and thighs

Working the muscles in your hips and thighs increases mobility, and helps to stabilize and balance your pelvis and hip area. Another advantage is that it will help make you look slimmer.

INTRODUCTION

Unless you were born with a figure to rival that of a supermodel, you probably wish your lower half was slimmer and trimmer. The trouble is that hips and thighs are often hard to target—for example, the muscles in your legs are much bigger than those in your arms, so you need to put more effort into getting results.

The benefits

General exercise such as running isn't always effective, so the great thing about this section is that each and every one of the exercises focuses entirely on slimming down and toning up these two trouble zones.

As you can imagine, most involve a lot of leg work and it may take some time for you to build up enough strength in the legs to be able to carry out the series of exercises outlined in the program, but with practice it will get easier.

Why not take your hip and thigh measurements before you start the plan and again when you finish? Seeing a reduction will spur you on and give you a great sense of achievement.

A HELPING HAND FOR HIPS AND THIGHS

For slimmer thighs and hips, follow a low-fat diet in addition to your toning and shaping routines.

• Trim all visible fat off meat.

• Steam or grill food rather than frying or boiling.

• Fill up with carbohydrates that release their energy slowly—for example, whole grain pasta, rice and cereals.

• Eat plenty of fresh fruit and vegetables.

• Drink plenty of water. This will flush out toxins from your body that can cause the appearance of dimpled flesh on your thighs.

Effective exercising

Most of these muscle-building exercises are done as a series of repetitions. For exercises that need repeating in order to last for 30 seconds, simply do as many repetitions as you can comfortably achieve in that time. The aim of repeating exercises is to work until your muscles feel tired, and over time this will strengthen them so that they can work even harder. To make it effective, it's important that you don't stop for more than a minute between exercises. Shorter recovery periods result in better muscles all round and improved muscle endurance. So keep going!

What you'll need

For this section you'll need a non-slip mat or pair of trainers, a chair, two tennis balls, a platform to step up on to or a sturdy bottom stair on a staircase, ankle weights (optional), and a cushion. Don't forget to warm up before you begin and cool down when you finish.

Now let's get started.

POSTURE

Practice these easy exercises to improve your posture. Remember to keep your movements smooth and flowing throughout.

Backside tilt

This simple exercise works your hip extensors (gluteus maximus) and is essential for good posture.

1 Stand up straight with your feet hip-width apart and your knees slightly bent. Rest your hands on the top of your hips.

2 Tighten your abdominal muscles by gently pulling in your navel toward your spine—don't suck in your waist or hold your breath.

3 Slowly tilt your pelvis forward then return to the starting position. The movement should come from your buttocks.

4 Slowly tilt your pelvis backward then return to the starting position.

5 Aim to do around six to eight.

4

Up and down

This is a good exercise for strengthening the quadriceps and for improving your body's alignment. You'll need two small balls for this exercise—tennis balls are ideal.

1 Stand behind a chair and place one ball between your ankles. Place the other ball between your legs just above your knees. Hold on to the chair to keep your balance.

2 Stand up straight with good posture. Slowly rise up on your toes.

3 Slowly come back down again. When your heels are on the floor, gently bend your knees, keeping your heels on the ground. Slowly move up into the starting position.

4 Aim to do around six to ten.

2

WATCH POINT

Don't bend forward or backward as you bend your knees.

STANDING EXERCISES 1

If you only ever do one type of hip and thigh exercise, make it a squat, which really hits the spot! Squats work the hip extensors, hamstrings (back of thigh muscles) and quadriceps (front of thigh muscles). Tight quads and hamstrings cause poor posture and lower back pain so it's very important to keep them in good working order.

Basic squat

Targeting the buttocks and the thighs, this easy exercise is great for toning up those trouble spots. Remember to keep your knees soft (slightly bent) throughout.

1 Stand up with good posture, your feet hip-width apart and your hands on your hips.

2 Tighten your abdominal muscles by gently pulling your navel toward your spine.

3 Bend your knees and squat as if you were going to sit down. Only squat as far as is comfortable and without losing your balance.

4 Return to the standing position by pushing through your heels, keeping your knees slightly bent.

5 Aim to do around eight to twelve.

Single-leg squat

This slightly harder squat really challenges your balance as well as working your hips and thigh muscles.

1 Standing with your feet together and your arms by your sides, shift your weight on to your right foot. Rest the toes of your left foot next to your right foot for balance.

2 Keeping your back straight, bend at the hips and knees and slowly sit back on to your right leg, raising your arms in front of you as you lower. Sit back only as far as is comfortable. Stop and hold for a count of two.

3 Now press into your right foot through the heels and come back up.

4 Repeat the exercise with the weight on your left foot.

5 Aim to do around six to ten.

2

WATCH POINT

Keep your abdominal muscles tight throughout these exercises.

SEATED EXERCISES

Even if you're office-bound for a large part of the day or spend a lot of time travelling, you can still sneak in a few exercises to keep your hips and thigh muscles toned. You'll need a straight-backed, sturdy chair for these exercises—not one on castors.

Seated leg extension

This easy exercise is great for toning the quadriceps, the muscles at the front of your thighs. To make this harder, you can use ankle weights to strengthen the intensity of the exercise.

1 Sit up straight with good posture. Tighten your abdominal muscles by pulling in your navel toward your spine—this will protect your back muscles.

2 Press your knees together and straighten one leg. Hold and release. Do all your repetitions on one leg, then repeat on the other leg.

3 Aim to do around six for each leg.

Simple seated thigh squeeze

This tones and strengthens your inner thighs. Make this exercise harder by increasing the time of the squeeze and by using something with more resistance, such as a semi-inflated ball.

1 Sit up straight on a chair with your knees bent and feet together.

2 Place a cushion between your thighs. Squeeze the cushion as hard as possible for a count of five, then release.

3 Aim to do around six.

2

MAKING THE EFFORT

It's important to work at the right intensity if you're aiming to tone up your muscles—if you work out until it hurts you may damage your muscles; put in too little effort and you won't notice any difference. Muscle soreness and stiffness is highly likely in the beginning, but if you can hardly move then you've overdone it. Rest up for a day or so and start again at a reduced intensity.

FLOOR EXERCISES 1

As well as tightening up your gluteals, these bridging exercises will help to stabilize your pelvis and your trunk muscles, and work your hamstrings. Take care not to over-arch your back or let it sag, and remember to keep your breathing steady and controlled throughout.

Stability bridge

You need to perfect this exercise in order to improve the stability of the trunk muscles before you can move on to more challenging movements.

1 Lie on your back with your knees bent and your feet flat on the floor, slightly apart. Keep your arms by your sides, palms facing downward.

2 Tighten your abdominal muscles by gently drawing in your navel toward your spine.

3 Press your lower back down into the floor and gently tilt your pelvis forward so that the pubic bone rises.

4 Use your hip, thigh and trunk muscles to lift your pelvis until your body forms a straight line from your shoulders to your knees. Hold for a count of five then return to the starting position.

5 Aim to do around two to four.

4

Bridge with leg lift

Lifting one leg strengthens the muscles at the back of the buttocks and thighs while increasing balance and control in your stabilizing muscles.

1 Lie on your back with your knees bent and feet slightly apart, and your arms at your sides.

2 Tighten your abdominal muscles by gently drawing in your navel toward your spine.

3 Curl your bottom off the floor, lifting your pelvis until your knees, hips and chest are in line.

4 Extend one leg, lift it level with the knee then lower to the floor. Do all your repetitions on one leg, then repeat on the other leg.

5 Aim to do around six to eight for each leg.

CONTROLLING YOUR MOVEMENTS

If an action hurts or you do it too quickly then you're not doing it properly. Movements should flow in a gentle, controlled manner. This enables your muscles to stretch naturally.

4

STANDING EXERCISES 2

As well as exercising your hip and thigh muscles, these leg lifts help to improve your balance. You will need to hold on to the back of a chair or a table for support for all these exercises. Keep movements smooth and fluid and move only as far as is comfortable.

Lateral leg raise

This exercise helps to tone and tighten your outer thigh muscles and your hips, as well as improve your balance.

1 Stand up straight with good posture, hands by your sides and feet together, holding on to the back of a chair with both hands for balance.

2 Tighten your abdominal muscles by gently drawing in your navel toward your spine. This will protect your lower back muscles.

3 Raise one leg out to the side about 45 degrees. Keep your toes pointing forward and hold for a count of three. Relax and do all your repetitions on one leg, then repeat using the other leg.

4 Aim to do around ten to twelve for each leg.

3

WATCH POINT

Keep your body straight and both knees soft throughout.

Front leg raise

This exercise strengthens and tones the front of your thighs (quadriceps) and increases your hip flexibility. It also helps with your balance.

1 Stand up straight with your feet together and hold on to the back of a chair sideways with your left hand to balance. Tighten your stomach muscles.

2 With your left leg slightly bent, raise your right leg out in front of you as far as is comfortable. Hold for a count of three.

3 Lower your leg, then do all your repetitions on that leg. Repeat on the other leg.

4 Aim to do around eight to twelve raises for each leg.

2

Rear leg raise

This strengthens and tones the buttocks, lower back, back of hips and hamstrings. It also helps with your balance. For best results, keep your buttocks tensed throughout—it's harder but better for you in the long run.

1 Stand up straight with your feet together and use your right hand to hold on to the back of a chair sideways to help you balance.

2 Pull in your stomach muscles to support your back and tighten your buttock muscles.

3

3 Take your right leg back, and touch the floor with your toes. Hold this position for a count of three, then return to the start. Do all your repetitions on one leg, then repeat on the other leg.

4 Aim to do around eight to twelve for each leg.

One-legged knee bends

These will strengthen your buttocks, thigh muscles and calves.

1 Stand up with good posture with your right side to the back of a chair and hold on to it for support. Lift and bend your right leg backward so that the knee faces forward and your foot is pointing out behind you in line with your knee.

2 Tighten your abdominal muscles to protect your back.

3 Slowly rise up on to the toes of your left foot. Hold for a count of two.

4 Slowly come back down again on to your left foot.

5 Now bend your left knee, bringing the kneecap directly over your foot.

6 Straighten up and repeat five times on the same leg, then do this exercise on the other leg.

7 Aim to do around six to eight for each leg.

3

WATCH POINT

Don't let your bottom stick out.

FLOOR EXERCISES 2

Make sure you perform each move slowly and in a controlled way to really work the muscles. You don't have to tense your buttocks as you do this but it's good to work your gluteals whenever you can.

Outer thigh lift

This exercise works the abductor muscles at the side of the thighs. Remember to keep your back straight, your hips facing forward, and breathe regularly throughout.

1 Lie on your right side with your body in a straight line and your thighs and feet together. Prop yourself up with your right arm and rest your left hand on the floor in front of you. Tighten your stomach muscles by drawing your navel in toward your spine—this will help protect your back.

2 Bend both knees. Lift up the top leg, then lower, squeezing your buttocks together as you raise and lower your leg.

3 Do all your repetitions on one side then repeat them on the other side of your body.

4 Aim to do around six to eight for each leg.

WATCH POINT

Keep the knee of the extended leg soft (slightly bent).

2

Inner thigh lift

This side-lying exercise works your inner thigh muscles (abductors). Remember to keep your spine in neutral and your stomach muscles tightened throughout.

1 Lie on one side with your hips facing forward and your body in a straight line. Prop yourself up on your elbow with your head resting on your hand and place the other hand on the floor in front of you for support.

2 Tighten your stomach muscles by gently drawing in your navel toward your spine to protect your back. Bend your top leg so that the knee touches the floor in front of you.

3 Raise the bottom extended leg, keeping the knee soft (slightly bent), then lower.

4 Do all your repetitions on one side then repeat them on the other side of your body.

5 Aim to do around six to eight for each leg.

1

4

STRETCHES

Stretching relieves the muscle tension that is created by exercise and allows the muscles to relax to their full length. This ensures that their full range is used and they do not remain in a semi-contracted state. Stretches help to develop flexibility and keep your body supple and injury-free, and you can perform these at the end of your session, when your muscles are well warmed up.

Lying buttock stretch

This will stretch your buttocks and your thigh muscles.

1 Lie on your back and bend your legs. Cross your right ankle over your left knee and lift your left leg off the floor. You will feel a stretch on the outside thigh and buttock of your left leg.

2 Take hold of your left thigh with both hands and slowly draw the left knee in toward you. You will feel the stretch intensify.

3 Hold the stretch for a count of ten. Release and repeat on the other leg.

Lying quad stretch

1 Lie prone (face down) on the floor. Bend one knee and take hold of the foot of that leg with your hand and gently pull the foot toward your buttock.

2 Press your hip down toward the floor (which will ensure you stretch fully the quadriceps muscle that crosses the hip joint).

3 Hold the stretch for a count of ten, then release and repeat on the other leg.

Lying hamstring stretch

1 Lie on your back with your knees bent and your feet resting flat on the floor.

2 Lift one leg and grasp the back of the thigh with your hands.

3 Gently pull that leg toward your chest as far as is comfortable. Repeat on the other leg.

Sitting inner thigh stretch

It is very important to stretch the inner thigh (adductor) muscles because they help the quadriceps and hip flexors during running.

1 Sit on the floor with your knees bent and the soles of the feet together, keeping your back straight. Rest your hands on your inner thighs, just above your knees.

2 Use your arms to press downward to abduct the hip joints and thus stretch the inner thigh muscles as far as is comfortable. Hold for a count of 20, then release.

2

Sitting outer thigh stretch

1 Sit on the floor with your legs stretched out. Cross the left leg over the right leg, with the left foot flat on the floor on the outer side of the right knee.

4 Hold for a count of ten and feel the stretch in the top of the outer left hip region, then release. Repeat the exercise on the other side.

2 Rest your left hand on the floor behind your body, with your arm straight to support your upper body.

3 With your right hand, pull your left knee gently over to the right.

3

7 DAY PLAN

Here's a simple plan for you to follow, which should be repeated for a further week, making a full 14 day fitness program. Although these are broken down into 6-minute routines, if you're new to exercise don't feel you have to start off doing the whole routine—you can build up the amount of time you spend and the types of exercises you do. You can also make up your own routines.

The routines shown here will give your abdominal muscles a good workout. Each routine should take 6 minutes to do, although this may vary depending on the amount of repetitions you do—don't worry if you can't do the full amount at first. The routines also take into account the time it will take for you to get into position and have a short rest between each exercise. The exercises in this book will tone your stomach muscles quickly, but be aware that they are not for fitness or weight loss.

Day 1

Backside tilt p108
Basic squat p110
Front leg raise p117
Rear leg raise p118
Outer thigh lift p120
Lying buttock stretch p122
Lying quad stretch p123
Lying hamstring stretch p123

Day 2

Seated leg extension p112
Simple seated thigh squeeze p113
Stability bridge p114
Bridge with leg lift p115
Lateral leg raise p116
Lying buttock stretch p122
Sitting inner thigh stretch p124

Day 3

Up and down p109
Seated leg extension p112
Outer thigh lift p120
Inner thigh lift p121
Lying buttock stretch p122
Sitting inner thigh stretch p124
Sitting outer thigh stretch p125

Day 4

Basic squat p110
Lateral leg raise p116
Front leg raise p117
Rear leg raise p118
One-legged knee bends p119
Lying buttock stretch p122
Lying quad stretch p123
Lying hamstring stretch p123

Day 5

Stability bridge p114
Bridge with leg lift p115
Outer thigh lift p120
Inner thigh lift p121
Lying buttock stretch p122
Sitting inner thigh stretch p124
Sitting outer thigh stretch p125

Day 6

Up and down p109
Basic squat p110
Lateral leg raise p116
Front leg raise p117
Rear leg raise p118
Lying buttock stretch p122
Lying quad stretch p123
Lying hamstring stretch p123

Day 7

Up and down p109
Single leg squat p111
One-legged knee bends p119
Outer thigh lift p120
Inner thigh lift p121
Lying buttock stretch p122
Lying quad stretch p123
Sitting inner thigh stretch p124
Sitting outer thigh stretch p125

EXERCISE INDEX